Frequently Asked Questions

all about
vitamins

JACK CHALLEM

AVERY PUBLISHING GROUP

Garden City Park • New York

The information contained in this book is based upon the research and personal and professional experiences of the author. They are not intended as a substitute for consulting with your physician or other health care provider. Any attempt to diagnose and treat an illness should be done under the direction of a health care professional.

The publisher does not advocate the use of any particular health care protocol, but believes the information in this book should be available to the public. The publisher and author are not responsible for any adverse effects or consequences resulting from the use of any of the suggestions, preparations, or procedures discussed in this book. Should the reader have any questions concerning the appropriateness of any procedure or preparation mentioned, the author and the publisher strongly suggest consulting a professional health care advisor.

ISBN: 0-89529-875-9

Printed in the United States of America

10   9   8   7   6   5   4

Contents

Introduction

Vitamins. They captivate. And they cure. Few newspaper headlines grab our attention faster than those describing the often "miraculous" benefits of vitamins. Almost every week, we hear reports that they can cure heart disease, ease the aches and pains of arthritis, and reduce the risk of cancer. Vitamins sound almost too good to be true. But are they as good as we've been told?

The answer, in a nutshell, is a resounding *yes*. For years, many doctors dismissed the value of vitamins, preferring to prescribe more expensive drugs or to perform surgery. Now, each year, medical journals publish thousands of scientific articles detailing the health benefits of vitamins, minerals, and other nutrients. And over the past ten years, more doctors have become tuned into vitamins.

Vitamins have many advantages over drugs. They're natural substances that work with your body to promote health. They're safe and relatively inexpensive. They help keep you well. They work.

But with all of the research on vitamins, it's also easy to become overwhelmed and confused. *All About Vitamins* is designed to clear the confusion by providing simple, straightforward answers to your questions about vitamins. In Chapter 1, you'll learn some vitamin "basics," including why vitamins are so important to your health and why supplements are necessary even if you're eating a healthy diet. Following this, each chapter answers your questions about one specific vitamin or family of vitamins: vitamin A, the B vitamins, and vitamins C, D, E, and K. There is even information on nutrients that function like vitamins. And the last chapter offers important tips on how to buy and use vitamins. A simple glossary of terms has been provided so that you can easily understand not only this book, but also other materials that you choose to read on this topic. And if you're interested in learning more about vitamins, you'll find that a helpful reading list has been included.

Read on. And be well.

1.

What Vitamins Can Do for Your Health

Your body requires relatively small amounts of vitamins compared with the other types of nutrients that are found in foods. Still, many people do not obtain enough vitamins, either because they don't eat the right foods or because they have absorption problems. Low levels of vitamins interfere with health. Unfortunately, many people go through life believing that health problems due to vitamin deficiencies are simply a normal part of life or aging. When such people take vitamin supplements for the first time, they discover just how dramatically vitamins can improve health. This chapter addresses the most basic issues regarding vitamins and health.

Q. What exactly are vitamins?

A. Vitamins are organic compounds (that is, compounds that contain at least one carbon atom) that function as coenzymes and cofactors that initiate and promote virtually all biochemical processes in the body. Your body cannot make most vitamins, or at least not in substantial amounts, so you have to obtain them from foods or supplements.

The thirteen essential vitamins are divided into two groups. One group consists of water-soluble vitamins, which need to be replenished daily because they are rapidly excreted. These vitamins include vitamin C and the B-complex family of vitamins. The second group consists of fat-soluble vitamins, which the body is capable of storing for weeks or months. The fat-soluble vitamins are vitamins A, D, E, and K. There are also a number of "vitamin-like" nutrients, such as beta-carotene, lutein, lycopene, coenzyme Q_{10}, and alpha-lipoic acid. These nutrients don't meet the strict definition of vitamins, but they are a lot like vitamins in what do they and how they work.

Q. What can vitamins do for me?

A. Whether you're young or old, male or female, work hard physically or have a desk job, vitamin supplements can have an almost miraculous effect on your health. Vitamins are one of several types of nutrients that serve as the building blocks of your body and its biochemicals. (The other building-block nutrients are protein, carbohydrates, fats, and minerals.) In a sense, vitamins help maintain the very structure of your heart, lungs, skin, brain, and other organs. They are also ingredients in the chemicals your body needs to make enzymes, hormones, energy, and new cells such as blood or skin cells. Basically, you need vitamins and minerals to grow, produce energy, fight disease, repair injured tissue, and maintain normal health. Because they help your body work the way it's supposed to, vitamins can help reduce your risk of developing such serious diseases as heart disease, cancer, and arthritis.

Properly supplementing vitamins will help your body not only to function well, but to function *optimally*. A recent study found that vitamin E supplements dramatically decrease the risk of coronary heart disease. Other studies have found that vitamin C reduces symptoms of the common cold and flu by one-third, basically meaning that the vitamin cuts your sick time by a couple of days. Still other studies have found that high intakes of vitamins lower the risk of many different types of cancer. In fact, many doctors are now turning to vitamins to treat diseases and to prevent diseases in their patients.

One of the most amazing things that occurs with vitamin supplementation is what Ron Hunninghake, MD, of Wichita, Kansas, calls "side benefits." In his medical practice, Hunninghake often finds that a vitamin supplement prescribed for one condition, such as arthritis, produces unexpected benefits, such as improvements in sleep or mood.

Recent research shows that many vitamins also influence the behavior of genes in a positive way. (So much for inheriting "bad" genes!) Vitamins protect genes from damage, "turn on" good genes, and "turn off" bad genes. The proper functioning of your genes is important because they control your health and your risk of developing cancer. So by helping your body to continue its normal functioning, vitamins promote health and prevent disease.

Q. Can vitamins reverse my health problems?

A. Can water quench thirst? Of course it can. Similarly, vitamin supplements can correct and reverse many long-standing health problems. As an example, British researchers recently conducted a study on individuals who had suffered heart attacks. Some of the men and women were given natural vitamin E supplements (400 to 800 IU daily), while others were given dummy pills. After an average of eighteen months, the participants who were getting vitamin E had 77 percent fewer additional heart attacks than those given the dummy pills.

Here's another example. Abram Hoffer, MD, PhD, of Victoria, Canada, has been treating terminal cancer patients with a high-potency vitamin/mineral regimen. Thirty percent of his early cancer patients, considered long-term users of supplements, were alive ten years after prognosis had predicted they wouldn't be. So the answer is *yes*, vitamins can reverse very serious diseases. You'll read about Hoffer's regimen later in this book.

Q. Are vitamin supplements safe?

A. Vitamin supplements are extraordinarily safe. There are only two vitamins—vitamins A and D—that pose some risk in very high doses, because the body stores them. However, it is much more common that people are deficient in these vitamins, rather than that they overdose on them.

In general, it's important to follow the usage directions given on the bottles of vitamins. Such directions will typically recommend RDA (Recommended Dietary Allowance) levels for vitamins A and D. (The RDA for vitamin A is 5,000 IU, and the RDA for vitamin D is 400 IU.) However, higher doses are often warranted. For example, a recent study, published in the *New England Journal of Medicine*, found that vitamin D deficiency was fairly common among people who, according to recommended standards, should have been getting enough of the vitamin.

There are ways to avoid putting yourself at risk of overdosing. For example, vitamin A in the form of beta-carotene is safe; the body converts beta-carotene to vitamin A as it's needed. You'll read more about the appropriate uses of high-dose vitamins A and D later in this book.

Q. Vitamins seem to do what a lot of drugs do. Are vitamin supplements drugs?

A. No, vitamin supplements are not drugs. They are natural substances that would normally be obtained through the diet. But because of poor eating habits, such as consuming too many junk foods and too few fruits and vegetables, many people do not obtain enough vitamins. So supplements are important.

In supplement form, vitamins work by promoting and supplying necessary nutrition for normal biological processes. In contrast, drugs work by *interfering* with natural processes in the body. Your body naturally needs vitamins, while it doesn't naturally need drugs. Think about this: you don't develop a headache because of an aspirin deficiency. However, there are scientific reports showing that vitamin B_2 deficiency can sometimes cause migraine headaches.

Q. Why don't more doctors recommend vitamin supplements?

A. "In medicine, doctors generally hold the view that vitamins are not real medicines," observes Richard Kunin, MD, of San Francisco. He continues, "Almost all medical minds have not been taught that nutrients represent the most dynamic aspect of body chemistry." For a long time, conventional medicine turned to synthesized substances that were not natural to the body, and used these products to impose changes in health. But today, more and more doctors are taking and recommending vitamin supplements. The medical community is realizing that what is best for the body is what is natural for the body.

Other physicians, such as Peter Langsjoen, MD, a cardiologist in Tyler, Texas, point out that drug companies influence much of a physician's education after medical school. Drug companies are going to market and sell their products, not low-cost natural alternatives. A number of studies have found that physicians tend to prescribe what they hear about the most, just as the average shopper tends to buy the big brand names over the little ones. So if your doctor is not giving you suggestions on vitamin intakes for health management, he or she simply may not be familiar with how vitamin supplements can make a difference in your life.

Q. If I'm already healthy, why should I take vitamins?

A. *Prevention* of disease is the key to prolonged health, not reversing disease once it has attacked the body. You can prevent—or at least reduce the risk of—disease by eating a diet high in fruits and vegetables, by exercising, and by taking vitamin supplements. While vitamins can correct a lot of damage and reverse or slow the course of many diseases, it's far better to maintain a disease free body. If you're in really good health now, it may take a few years before you observe any obvious benefits from vitamin supplementation. But you'll probably notice that you don't get sick as often as people who aren't taking vitamins. Your cholesterol and blood pressure probably won't go up as much as theirs. You won't have as many aches and pains, and you'll have a good energy level.

Q. Don't I get enough vitamins in the food I eat?

A. Probably not—and there are several reasons for this. One is that many people don't select very nutritious foods. Fruits and vegetables are particularly high in most vitamins, and the U.S. Department of Agriculture recommends that people eat three to five servings of fruits and vegetables daily. But according to researchers at the University of California, Berkeley, only an estimated 9 percent of Americans consume adequate daily amounts of fruits and vegetables. Even the most optimistic study found that only one out of every three Americans ate three to five fruits and vegetables daily. It's easy to be tempted by burgers, fries, and fried chicken, to skip salads and broccoli, and, therefore, to miss a lot of vitamins.

Another reason people often don't get enough vitamins is that the staple foods of the American diet have undergone tremendous changes in processing over the past hundred years. In the nineteenth century, people ate whole-grain breads rich in vitamin E. Around 1900, technological changes in the milling of grains removed the vitamins, leaving white starch for bread-making. As if this weren't bad enough, food processing has promoted the use of cooking oils from grains (such as corn and soy oil), which increase our vitamin E requirements. In a sense, we're caught between a rock and a hard place, in terms of getting enough vitamins!

Furthermore, soils deficient in some minerals limit a plant's production of vitamins. Synthetic fertilizers (in contrast to plain old manure) don't solve the problem. Several years ago, U.S. Department of Agriculture researchers found that conventional nitrogen fertilizer reduces vitamin C levels in some food crops by as much as one-third. Additional nutrient losses have been documented during the transportation, storage, and processing of produce, as well as during cooking. So even if your intentions are good, it's often hard to buy and prepare adequately nutritious foods.

Q. Is the average diet really that bad?

A. Despite official proclamations that Americans have the best food supply in the world, a large number of Americans don't obtain sufficient amounts of the essential nutrients. Nutritional surveys have found that 50 percent of Americans consume less than 50 mg of vitamin C daily, while 25 percent consume less than 39 mg. These intakes fall far below the Recommended Dietary Allowance (RDA) of 60 mg. Other studies have found that half of the population consumes only 950 IU of vitamin A (19 percent of the RDA), and 4 IU of vitamin E (40 percent of the RDA) or less, daily. The same pattern applies to the consumption of other vitamins and minerals as well, meaning that large numbers of people aren't getting adequate nutrition.

Unfortunately, even a good diet and healthy supplementation cannot a guarantee that your body is doing a good job absorbing nutrients. I am very committed to eating a good diet and taking my vitamins. According to an analysis of my diet, I was eating RDA levels of nearly everything. But when I recently had a physician do a comprehensive nutritional work-up on me, my blood tests showed a different picture. Among other things, my vitamin B_1 levels were one-third of normal, even though I was taking about thirty times the RDA of this vitamin. So a standard healthy regimen may not be giving you what you need. The safest bet is to have a nutritional program designed specifically for you.

Q. A lot of foods, such as the cereals I eat, contain 100 percent of the RDA for vitamins. How come this isn't enough?

A. As stated before, each person has his or her own nutrient requirements. You may not be getting enough of certain vitamins, even though your intakes match the guidelines of the RDAs. Actually, many physicians and researchers consider the RDA an outdated and conservative dietary standard. If that's the case, people malnourished by RDA standards are in very bad shape. If they were cars, they'd be driving on fumes.

The predecessor to today's RDA was designed by the federal government as a guideline for "practically all healthy persons" during World War II. But many prominent nutrition researchers have questioned whether Americans can be considered healthy and, therefore, whether RDA levels of vitamins are really adequate. For example, Paul LaChance, PhD, of Rutgers University, has pointed out that 30 percent of Americans smoke, and many drink too much alcohol. Countless people suffer from diabetes, high cholesterol levels, and hypertension. An article in the *Journal of the American Medical Association* recently reported that 45 percent of Americans suffer from at least one chronic condition. "After age 45, most people are not 'healthy' in the strict sense of the word and relatively few qualify as having no chronic or acute problem," LaChance recently explained in the journal *Nutrition Reviews*.

For example, vitamin B_6, folic acid (another B vitamin), and vitamin E are three of the vitamins most important for a healthy heart. A study by Harvard University researchers found that folic acid and vitamin B_6 protect against coronary heart disease. However, the most beneficial dose was three or more times the RDA. Similarly, vitamin E seems to offer the most protection to the heart at 400 IU daily—forty times the RDA.

By the way, don't be scared off by a product that contains 400 percent of the RDA. This amount is four times, not 400 times, the RDA.

Q. Is it true that some people need more vitamins than others?

A. You have probably heard the phrase, "One man's meat is another's poison." What works for one person may not work for another. This is true for vitamin supplementation as well. The very concept of an RDA may be flawed.

In the 1950s (yes, a very long time ago), Roger Williams, PhD, who discovered the B-vitamin pantothenic acid, developed the concept of *biochemical individuality*. Basically, biochemical individuality refers to the fact that we are all nutritional individuals. Williams found that people need the same basic groups of vitamins and other nutrients, but that they are highly individualistic in the required amounts for optimal health benefits. For one person, 100 mg daily of vitamin C might be sufficient for health, while for another, 3,000 mg would be most effective.

These differences stem from our genetic individuality. Peoples' stomachs come in all shapes and sizes, and some people produce far more digestive enzymes than others. The person with good digestion will absorb nutrients better than the person with poor digestion. These differences exist on a very minute level in the body, but they have profound effects on our health and the likelihood of disease. So the bottom line is that everyone needs vitamins, but different people need different vitamins in different amounts. One size does not fit all.

Q. I'm a vegetarian and I eat a good diet. Do I need to take vitamins?

A. If you're a vegetarian, you've got a lot going in your favor, but adequate vitamins levels aren't guaranteed through your diet. In general, vegetarians enjoy better health than meat-eaters. One study, published in the *British Medical Journal*, found that vegetarians were far less likely than meat-eaters to die from heart disease, stroke, and cancer. There are two reasons for this: fruits and vegetables—the bulk of the vegetarian diet—provide a lot of vitamins, and conscientious vegetarians tend to avoid junk foods loaded with fats and sugars, which increase vitamin requirements. However, vegetarians may be lacking in some nutrients. A study in the *Journal of the American Dietetic Association* reported that female vegetarians tend to have lower levels of vitamins B_2, B_3, B_{12}, sodium, and zinc.

Q. Is there anyone who doesn't suggest taking vitamin supplements?

A. Yes. Some organizations, such as the American Dietetic Association, routinely state that people should get all of the nutrients they need from a "balanced" diet. But according to Emanuel Cheraskin, MD, DMD, professor emeritus at the University of Alabama, Birmingham, such a diet is not enough. Cheraskin has pointed out that today's world is hardly a natural environment, and thus a natural diet, by itself, cannot offer us full protection. He sees vitamin supplements as "heroic countermeasures" against this unnaturally polluted and stressful environment. For example, vitamin C boosts the production of compounds in your liver that help detoxify hazardous chemicals, such as those lurking in air pollution.

Q. How good is the scientific research on vitamins?

A. The scientific research supporting the roles of vitamins in health is far better than the research on most drugs. On average, journals publish about 500 to 600 studies a year on vitamin E, and about an equal number on vitamin C. Recently, over the past five years, medical and scientific journals around the world have published more than 5,000 articles on antioxidants, which include vitamins C and E and closely related vitamin-like nutrients. If you review this research, you'll notice two clear trends, regardless of whether the studies are on people, animals, or cells. One trend is that higher levels of vitamins and minerals are almost always associated with health. The other trend is that lower levels of these nutrients are almost always associated with disease.

Also important is the fact that research techniques advance with time. In the 1940s and 1950s, when a handful of physicians started using vitamins to treat disease, no one really understood how these nutrients worked. Today, researchers have gained a better explanation of how vitamins and minerals function. For example, vitamin E helps the cardiovascular system by maintaining normal blood vessel flexibility, reducing the heart-damaging effects of cholesterol, and blocking the activity of disease-promoting compounds. So the body of research on vitamins has become more and more informative.

Q. What are free radicals?

A. Free radicals are a big reason why people get old and develop degenerative diseases. To understand how free radicals do their damage, you'll have to learn a little (only one paragraph's worth) about atoms and electrons.

The basic building blocks of all matter consist of atoms. Each atom has electrons circling it, in much the same way that the moon circles the earth. Normally, electrons come in pairs. When an atom is short one electron, or has one too many, it's called a *free radical*. The radical is "free" in the sense that it's cruising around aggressively and looking for a mate. If it picks up a replacement electron from an atom that's part of your deoxyribonucleic acid (DNA, or genetic material), it will damage the DNA in the process. Oxygen, which you need to breathe, is the source of most free radicals, so the damage caused by free radicals is called *oxidation*.

Free radical oxidation is what makes butter turn rancid and iron get rusty. In your body, it leads impaired DNA to replicate the damages, and this leads to cell abnormalities and aging. When oxidation occurs in enough of your cells, your body ages and your risk of cancer and other diseases increases.

Although free radicals are found in cigarette smoke and other pollutants, they are also a byproduct of normal cellular processes. For example, the body produces free radicals to kill infectious bacteria. Too much exposure to sunlight also generates free radicals, which is why sun worshippers tend to have older looking skin.

Q. Antioxidants are always discussed along with free radicals. What are antioxidants—vitamins?

A. Antioxidants, when compared with free radicals, are the flip side of the coin, because they quench (or neutralize) free radicals. Many vitamins and vitamin-like nutrients function as antioxidants and, in doing so, they limit cellular damage. Vitamins E and C are antioxidants, as are beta-carotene, lutein, coenzyme Q_{10}, and alpha-lipoic acid.

There is supposed to be somewhat of a balance in the body between free radicals and antioxidants, since both are needed for health. However, according to Lester Packer, PhD, a leading biologist at the University of California, Berkeley, trouble begins when there are too many free radicals, which leads to oxidation and "oxidative stress." Too many free radicals promote inflammation and degenerative diseases. This is where antioxidant vitamins help restore balance.

Q. Can I get by with taking just one antioxidant?

A. While your health will certainly benefit from simply taking vitamin E or vitamin C, you'll do much better by taking a combination of antioxidants. Researcher Al L. Tappel, PhD, of the University of California, Davis, has shown that a diverse selection of antioxidants may be more important than high doses of just one or two. That doesn't mean you have to swallow handfuls of antioxidant tablets and capsules. For reducing your long-term risk of disease, consider taking an antioxidant "cocktail" containing four to ten different antioxidants. If you're already taking a high-potency multivitamin, you may be getting enough antioxidants.

Q. Can vitamins really keep me young?

A. Aging is the result of damage to the 100 trillion cells that compose your body. The net effect is that these cells become less and less efficient with age. An old heart doesn't pump blood as well as a young heart. An old stomach doesn't digest food as well as a young stomach. To use an analogy, vitamins are like biological spark plugs that energize your cells and also protect them. They promote the myriad biological activities of your cells and, in doing so, they keep them functioning more like younger cells. This isn't just theory, by the way. Numerous studies have shown that vitamin supplements extend life expectancy. Inadequate intake of vitamins decreases life expectancy.

Q. I've heard the term *orthomolecular* nutrition or medicine. What does it mean?

A. The term *orthomolecular*, coined by the late Nobel laureate Linus Pauling, PhD, literally means "to straighten out molecules." Orthomolecular nutrition and medicine aim to use natural nutrients and chemicals to restore proper balance in the body, thus reversing and preventing disease. Pauling, regarded second only to Einstein when it comes to twentieth-century scientists, saw life in largely molecular terms. Instead of suggesting RDA levels of nutrients, which aim at vitamin adequacy, Pauling believed that people should think in terms of optimal levels of vitamins. He spent the last thirty years of his life researching vitamin C (among other things) and contended that people should take at least 1 g (1,000 mg) of vitamin C daily. He himself took 18 g daily, but most people probably don't need quite that much.

Q. So, do I have to take "megadoses" of some vitamins?

A. A megadose, like beauty, is really in the eyes of the beholder. Dietitians, who are notoriously conservative when it comes to supplements, tend to feel that anything above the RDA level constitutes a megadose. However, the trend in nutrition research is toward developing recommendations that are higher than the current RDAs.

A growing number of researchers and physicians believe that vitamin levels that amount to roughly three times the RDA are often optimal doses. In an experiment, Mark Levine, MD, PhD, of the National Institutes of Health at Bethesda, Maryland, found that 200 mg of vitamin C daily—more than three times the RDA—was the ideal intake for young, healthy men. But Levine's study didn't look at women or sick people (about half of the population), so he was reluctant to apply his recommendations to the general population.

Many others, particularly practicing physicians, have had great success treating patients with so-called megadoses of vitamins. Some of these doctors, such as Hugh Riordan, MD, of Wichita, Kansas, use laboratory tests to carefully document that patients who originally had low levels of vitamins showed marked improvement when taking high doses of vitamin supplements. Robert Cathcart III, MD, of Los Altos, California, recommends large amounts of vitamin C (and other vitamins and minerals) to patients with severe infections ranging from colds and flus to mononucleosis and AIDS.

"Taking megadoses is a really good thing to do if you want to stay alive," says Hyla Cass, MD, a psychiatrist in Pacific Palisades, California. "Our diets are terribly deficient in the nutrients we need to keep us alive and to function optimally. We're eating foods grown on mineral-depleted soils, and people are getting pesticides that interfere with absorption. The RDA is barely a survival amount, so we definitely need to supplement."

Q. Should I work with a physician in taking high doses of vitamins?

A. Nutritionally-oriented physicians customarily recommend that patients work with a specialized physician when it comes to treating a specific disease with nutritional changes and supplements. This is good advice, but many people don't follow it, perhaps because it's too hard to find a doctor who knows something about vitamins, or because their insurance won't reimburse them for the doctors' care. As a consequence, lots of people end up treating themselves with vitamins, which isn't really all that bad. Vitamins are very safe, and people have a right to treat themselves. (For example, vitamins are safer than aspirin, which many people take to treat headaches.) Still, you should, at the very least, let your doctor know that you're taking vitamins, even if he doesn't believe vitamins have any benefits. (You may have to assert yourself here and tell your doctor that you intend to take vitamins unless he can come up with a good reason why you shouldn't.)

Also, it's wise to read up on anything you take, whether it's a vitamin or a prescription drug. While this book is a starting point, there are others that go into more depth about vitamins and how to use them. Some of these books are listed in the suggested reading section toward the end of this book. You can buy many of them at book stores and health food stores, or you can borrow them from a public library.

Q. If I take a lot of vitamins in supplements, won't I just excrete them and have "expensive urine"?

A. This is one of the most common arguments used by doctors who ignore the research on vitamins and, sometimes, build their careers on being anti-vitamin curmudgeons. It's a foolish argument against vitamins, and here's why: If you drink an expensive bottle of wine, you'll also have expensive urine. Ditto for a prime steak—your body will use part of it, and turn the rest into expensive stools. Should you then eat and drink the cheapest foods possible? Of course not! You should eat the most nutritious foods possible.

Your body does not absorb 100 percent of any nutrient you eat. In fact, you absorb a relatively small portion of what you consume. It's no different with vitamins. When you take large doses of vitamins, your absorption becomes less efficient, but you'll still absorb more overall than if you took a smaller amount.

2.

Vitamin A and the Carotenoids

Vitamin A is an essential dietary nutrient found in animal foods, and the carotenoids are found in fruits and vegetables. Some of the carotenoids are closely related to vitamin A. For example, the human body converts some beta-carotene, one of the most common carotenoids, to vitamin A. But this is not true for all carotenoids; lutein and lycopene play important roles in health, but the body cannot convert them to vitamin A. Also, vitamin A has weak antioxidant activity, whereas beta-carotene, lutein, and lycopene are powerful antioxidants and carry out vitamin-like activities.

Q. I've always heard that vitamin A is good for the eyes. Is this true?

A. Yes, it is. Vitamin A is essential for vision. It helps convert light to signals your brain can "read," enabling you to see details and to distinguish colors. Inadequate intake of vitamin A causes *night blindness*. This is a condition in which the eyes have difficulty adjusting to the dark or to bright lights. Night blindness impairs the vision of the car driver in two ways. First, it limits the detail that he or she can see when it's dark. Second, it makes oncoming headlights seem brighter, causing the driver to be blinded by the glare. If it takes you more than a minute to adjust your eyes in a darkened theater, you probably have night blindness.

The treatment is relatively simple. The fastest way to correct night blindness is to increase your intake of vitamin A-containing foods, such as liver, or you can take daily supplements—25,000 IU daily for a month, then dropping down to 10,000 IU daily. You can also increase your intake of fruits and vegetables, or take beta-carotene capsules, but this approach will take longer than ingesting pure vitamin A.

Q. Can vitamin A help in retinitis pigmentosa?

A. Retinitis pigmentosa, or simply RP, is an inherited disease in which part of the eye's retina deteriorates prematurely. Night blindness can be an early sign of RP, but this disease also includes a narrowing of the visual field—kind of like looking through a tube. Ultimately, it leads to total blindness.

In a study by Harvard Medical School researchers, 15,000 IU of vitamin A daily greatly slowed the progression of RP. Based on the results of the study, a person with RP who begins taking vitamin A at the age of thirty-two will preserve some useful vision through the age of seventy—for seven years longer than he would if he hadn't been taking the vitamin. In addition, a preliminary study on the use of vitamin-like coenzyme Q_{10} found that 100 mg daily might improve some cases of RP. These two nutrients are certainly worth a try because there is no other treatment for RP.

Q. What else does vitamin A do?

A. Vitamin A is essential for the body's production of epithelial cells, which line most tissues and the skin. Many people find it helpful in skin disorders, such as cystic acne. When treating cystic acne, stick with the dosages recommended in this chapter.

One recent study found that a form of vitamin A might reverse emphysema, though the experiments so far have been limited to laboratory rats. Gloria De Carlo Massaro, MD, and Donald Massaro, MD, of the Georgetown University School of Medicine, Washington, DC, induced emphysema in the lungs of laboratory rats. Groups of lung cells called alveoli enlarged and turned hard. After the animals were given all-trans-retinoic acid—a form of vitamin A that the body makes from beta-carotene—production of normal alveoli increased by 50 percent.

Vitamin A also has hormone-like effects in that it controls the growth and normal differentiation of cells. What does this mean? Differentiation is a normal process that turns new cells into heart cells or lung cells or bone cells. Cancer cells are undifferentiated. In other words, vitamin A helps make normal cells.

Q. Will vitamin A help me fight off chest infections?

A. Back in 1928, in the *British Medical Journal*, leading nutrition researchers referred to vitamin A as the "anti-infective" vitamin. Vitamin A strengthens the epithelial cell barrier against attacking bacteria and viruses. When laboratory animals were deprived of vitamin A, they first lived in reasonably good health, but then took sudden and fatal turns. During autopsy, the researchers found extensive infections of the animals' internal organs. Thus, it was concluded that vitamin A helps to combat infection.

For years, children in developing nations were dying from measles, a respiratory disease that has been almost completely eliminated in Western nations. In the mid-1970s, Alfred Sommer, MD, of Johns Hopkins University, Baltimore, discovered that these children were severely deficient in vitamin A and that brief high-dose supplements could cut the death rate from measles by one-third. The preventive dosage is 100,000 IU of vitamin A daily for two days, followed by 100,000 IU one month later.

Some studies have shown high doses of vitamin A to be helpful in other respiratory infections, such as chicken pox and pneumonia. The key is high doses taken for a brief period of time, such as two days—not long-term, high-dose consumption.

Q. Are high doses of vitamin A toxic?

A. There is a remote risk of toxicity with vitamin A. That's why recommendations for treating respiratory (lung) infections are high doses for only two days. While the dose—100,000 IU—is very high, it's for too short a time to cause side effects, which include hair loss and headaches.

In general, it's quite safe for people to take 10,000 IU of vitamin A daily for years and years. Pregnant women, or women who plan to become pregnant, should probably take no more than 8,000 IU of vitamin A daily, because there is a slight risk of birth defects among pregnant women who take very large doses of this vitamin.

Q. What about beta-carotene—is it toxic in high doses as well?

A. No, beta-carotene is safe, even at very high doses. In some people, very high doses will turn the skin (particularly hands and feet) a yellow-orange color, but this is not dangerous and it goes away shortly after supplementation is stopped. Only a small portion of beta-carotene is converted to vitamin A, so you can't create toxic levels of vitamin A by taking a lot of beta-carotene.

Q. Beta-carotene is considered a carotenoid. What exactly are the carotenoids?

A. The carotenoids are fat-soluble antioxidants that plants produce to protect themselves from the damaging effects of free radicals, which are one of the basic causes of cancer, heart disease, and other degenerative diseases. More than 600 carotenoids are found in nature, though only about 50 are found in the Western diet. Of these, only 14 show up in the blood, indicating that they are absorbed. The principal dietary carotenoids appear to be beta-carotene (found in carrots), alpha-carotene (also found in carrots), lutein (found in kale, broccoli, and spinach), and lycopene (found in tomatoes). Other important, though minor, carotenoids are zeaxanthin and cryptoxanthin. When we eat foods containing carotenoids, we benefit from their antioxidant properties.

Q. What does beta-carotene specifically do?

A. In addition to being a source of vitamin A, beta-carotene quenches a type of free radical called *singlet oxygen*. Furthermore, several studies have reported that beta-carotene increases lung capacity—basically, the amount of oxygen you can breathe in and out. The more oxygen you can take in with a single breath, the healthier you are. Lung capacity generally decreases with age. Beta-carotene can help to combat this natural degeneration.

Q. Does beta-carotene increase the risk of cancer?

A. Two studies found that beta-carotene slightly increased the risk of lung cancer among current smokers, particularly if they also drank alcohol. But these studies used synthetic beta-carotene, which is different from the natural form found in supplements (which comes from *Dunaliella salina* algae) and does not contain a powerful natural antioxidant. Interestingly, one of these studies found that *former* smokers taking beta-carotene had a lower risk of developing lung cancer than those who didn't take it.

Many other studies have reported that beta-carotene, in combination with other antioxidants such as vitamin E and selenium, is good for health and actually anti-cancerous. Beta-carotene seems to work best as part of an antioxidant team, rather than by itself. However, beta-carotene supplements alone do not reverse *oral leukoplakia*, a precancerous condition found in smokers and drinkers.

Q. Can beta-carotene prevent me from sunburning?

A. It can. Several studies have found that a combination of beta-carotene supplements taken orally and conventional sunscreens applied to the skin work better than sunscreens alone. In a sense, beta-carotene helps provide inside-out protection against the ultraviolet (UV) radiation in sunlight. It most likely works by improving the skin's natural and internal defenses against UV damage.

This benefit directly contradicts the idea that beta-carotene might increase cancer risk. Excessive exposure to the sun damages the skin and increases the risk of skin cancer. By reducing damage to the skin, beta-carotene should reduce the long-term risk of UV-induced skin cancer. Other antioxidants, such as vitamins C and E, also help the skin to resist sunburn.

Q. Can beta-carotene do anything for my cholesterol?

A. Several studies have reported that beta-carotene can lower cholesterol levels a little. It seems to work, in part, by blocking the body's production of blood cholesterol. Other studies have found that beta-carotene has a modest effect in preventing the oxidation of, or free radical damage to, cholesterol. When cholesterol becomes oxidized, it seems to promote the development of coronary heart disease more than normal cholesterol does.

Q. Can the carotenoids help treat macular degeneration?

A. The *macula* is the center of the eye's retina (kind of like the screen in a theater), and its premature breakdown is the leading cause of blindness among Americans over the age of sixty-five. Two carotenoids seem to help preserve the macula. They are lutein and zeaxanthin. Together, they form the yellowish *macular pigment,* which filters out damaging ultraviolet light.

A study published in the *Journal of the American Medical Association* found that people eating foods rich in lutein—particularly kale and spinach—were less likely to develop macular degeneration. Several studies have reported that consuming lutein-rich foods or supplements increases the thickness of the macular pigment. Lutein supplements may not reverse macular degeneration, but researchers in this field believe they can slow down the progression of this disease. Zeaxanthin is also important to the macula, and it appears that the body can convert some lutein to zeaxanthin.

There is some evidence that lutein and zeaxanthin may also help retard the development of cataracts. Both of these carotenoids are found in the lens of the eye. But it's unclear whether or not they could reverse a cataract.

Q. Are the carotenoids good for the prostate?

A. Two carotenoids, lycopene and beta-carotene, seem to be. In a study in the *Journal of the National Cancer Institute*, Edward Giovannucci, MD, of Harvard University, reported that men eating large amounts of tomato sauces (more than ten servings weekly) were 45-percent less likely to develop prostate cancer. Raw tomatoes provided some benefit, while tomato juice didn't help at all.

Though the findings seem odd, there is a rationale behind them. Cooking tomatoes (for spaghetti or pizza sauces, for example) breaks down the cell walls containing lycopene, making more of this nutrient available for digestion and absorption. Such sauces are also made with olive oil, which aids lycopene absorption (because it is fat soluble). Raw tomatoes are typically eaten with either salad dressing or meat, so the oil or fat in these foods also aid absorption. Tomato juice is not cooked, nor does it contain additional oil.

Another Harvard University study found that among men not eating fruits and vegetables, beta-carotene supplements reduced the risk of prostate cancer by one-third. There was no additional benefit among men who were already eating their fruits and vegetables.

3.

The B Vitamin Family

The B vitamins—there are eleven of them—influence many different aspects of health, including energy level, mood and behavior, and risk of degenerative diseases such as heart disease and cancer. Some of the B vitamins, such as B_1, B_2, and B_3, play central roles in the conversion of food to energy. High doses of B_3 can often improve schizophrenia, a devastating mental disorder. Vitamin B_6 and folic acid can reduce the risk of heart disease. Read on to find out more information on how the B vitamins can improve your health.

Q. I've heard that the B vitamins are "anti-stress" vitamins. Is this true?

A. According to David Benton, PhD, a researcher and professor at the University of Swansea, Wales, the first signs of vitamin deficiencies appear as psychological problems. Among these problems are irritability, anger, and difficulty dealing with pressures at home or work. The B-complex vitamins have long been regarded as anti-stress vitamins. They are important for normal nerve and brain function, so inadequate levels of them will interfere with the nervous system.

To help deal with stress, start with a B-complex supplement. Look on the label to see if it contains 10 mg of vitamin B_1—this is a clue to the relative amounts of the other B vitamins in the supplement. If you don't sense any improvement after thirty days, either triple the dose or buy a B-complex supplement with 25 mg of vitamin B_1 (again, a clue to the amounts of other B vitamins).

You may find, as some doctors have pointed out, "side benefits" from such a supplement. For example, you may notice that your skin is in better condition. When I was in my twenties and suffering from dandruff, I happened to read that B vitamins might help with dry, flaky skin. I was already taking a 10-mg B-complex supplement, so I increased the dose, and my dandruff went away. I've continued taking my high-potency B-complex, and my dandruff has never returned.

Q. Can B vitamins improve my mood?

A. They certainly can. Consider the experiments

conducted by Benton. He gave some healthy students a high-potency multivitamin (containing ten times the RDA of most vitamins), while giving others placeboes (dummy pills) for a year. When he reevaluated the mood of the students, Benton found that the multivitamin group described themselves as more agreeable, and the women said their moods had improved significantly, according to his article in *Biological Psychology/Pharmacopsychology*.

Benton subsequently determined that while all of the vitamins seemed to help, vitamin B_1 stood out among the others. In a follow-up study, he gave female university students supplements of vitamin B_1. After just two months, the women described themselves as more clear-headed, self-composed, and energetic. They also had faster reaction times.

Q. Can the B vitamins ease migraine headaches?

A. Two recent studies show that vitamin B_2 may reduce the frequency of migraine headaches. In the first study, Jean Schoenen, MD, PhD, of the University of Liege, Belgium, treated forty-nine patients with 400 mg of B_2 daily, for three or more months. More than two-thirds of the patients improved. In the second study, Schoenen treated fifty-five patients, again giving them 400 mg of B_2 for three months. In this experiment, 59 percent of the patients on the supplements improved, compared with only 15 percent of those taking placeboes.

Q. Can the B vitamins lower my cholesterol?

A. Believe it or not, since 1955, the niacin (sometimes referred to as nicotinic acid) form of vitamin B_3 has been known to lower cholesterol. This was discovered by Abram Hoffer, MD, PhD, one of the pioneers in the medical use of vitamins. Other forms of vitamin B_3, such as niacinamide and nicotinamide, do not have this cholesterol-lowering effect. Hoffer recommends taking 500 mg of niacin, three times daily.

Before you take niacin, you should be aware of its principal side effect. After taking it, you will have a body-wide flushing or tingling sensation. Your skin will turn beet red and you'll feel itchy all over. All this is not harmful, but the reaction can be a little unsettling. The flushing sensation, which some people do like (it makes people feel warm), passes after about an hour. If you take niacin three times a day, and keep taking it day after day, this flushing reaction will lessen and stop.

Vitamin C supplements—1,000 mg daily—can also sometimes reduce blood cholesterol levels, without the flushing.

Q. Can any of the B vitamins help in the treatment of multiple sclerosis?

A. Multiple sclerosis is characterized by damage to the nerve sheaths or insulation. A number of studies have found that people with MS are consistently deficient in vitamin B_{12}. Low levels of folic acid may also be a problem. These two vitamins work hand in hand. However, many people have trouble absorbing B_{12} through the gut. Injections of B_{12} (from your doctor) get around this problem. So do sublingual tablets, which are small and meant to dissolve under the tongue (where absorption is very efficient).

In MS, it might also help to reduce your overall intake of fats and oils, while increasing your relative intake of the omega-3 fish oils and olive oil. In addition, increase your intake of antioxidants, such as vitamins E and C and alpha-lipoic acid. Pycnogenol, a natural complex of antioxidants from French maritime pine trees, might also help, due to its anti-inflammatory properties.

Q. Can the B vitamins relieve arthritis?

A. They probably can. Years ago, doctors found that they could ease symptoms of rheumatoid arthritis by giving one of the B vitamins, then ease symptoms some more by giving another B vitamin. It might be faster and more efficacious for you to simply take a high-potency B-complex supplement, rather than to try the B-vitamins one by one.

One study, reported in the *Journal of the American College of Nutrition,* found that supplements of folic acid (6,400 mcg) and vitamin B_{12} (20 mcg) relieved symptoms of osteoarthritis in the hands. A more recent study, in the German journal *Schmerz,* described the analgesic (pain-relieving) properties of vitamins B_1, B_2, and B_{12}. The researcher noted that the combination of these vitamins is more effective than individual supplementation.

Q. Can the B vitamins help with my PMS?

A. PMS (premenstrual syndrome) is often caused by excess estrogen, a female hormone. Two B vitamins, choline and inositol, help convert estrogen into estriol, a form of the hormone that doesn't seem to cause problems. In addition, vitamin B_6 is a diuretic and can prevent water retention before your menstrual period. If you take B_6 (50 to 100 mg daily), add a B-complex supplement for more optimal functioning.

Also, eating more soy foods should help normalize estrogen levels. Soybeans contain natural estrogen-like compounds that block the undesirable effects of the actual hormone. Soy milk, soy burgers, and tofu are a few types of the many soy foods available at your supermarket and health food store.

Q. Can the B vitamins help reduce carpal tunnel syndrome?

A. Carpal tunnel syndrome is characterized by extreme pain or numbness in the wrist and hand. It is caused by the stress of a repetitive motion of the hand, and supermarket cashiers, typists, and factory workers seem to be prone toward it.

Some thirty years ago, John Ellis, MD, of Mount Pleasant, Texas, found that vitamin B_6 could help patients with carpal tunnel syndrome. He concluded that patients with this disorder had low levels of vitamin B_6, and that taking 100 mg daily would restore normal levels after ninety days. Other researchers have also found strong associations between low vitamin B_6 levels and carpal tunnel syndrome. It's likely that the repetitive stress increases vitamin B_6 requirements.

It's unusual, however, for a person to be deficient in just one nutrient, and the B vitamins work together as a family of related nutrients. So a better regimen for carpal tunnel might be 100 mg of vitamin B_6, plus a B-complex supplement containing all of the members of this vitamin family.

Q. Does vitamin B help schizophrenia?

A. First, let's clarify what schizophrenia is. It is not a split personality. Rather, it is a mental disorder characterized by delusions (such as extreme paranoia) and hallucinations (seeing or hearing things that aren't there). In the early 1950s, Abram Hoffer, MD, PhD, and Humphry Osmond, MD, theorized that some types of schizophrenics produce a hallucinogen in their own bodies. The hallucinogen is an oxidized form of adrenaline.

Based on their knowledge of biochemistry, these doctors believed that high doses of vitamin B_3 (either niacin or niacinamide) and vitamin C would neutralize this hallucinogen. They turned out to be correct, and they published the first double-blind trial in the field of psychiatry in the *Bulletin of the Menninger Clinic.* In the late 1960s, when hallucinogenic drugs, such as LSD and mescaline, were popular, some people used vitamins B_3 and C to bring themselves down from "bad trips."

Hoffer tends to give schizophrenic patients 3,000 mg of vitamin B_3 and 1,000 to 3,000 mg of vitamin C daily. He has pointed out that patients with a recent onset of schizophrenia respond better to vitamin therapy than do patients who have suffered from schizophrenia for a very long time. Also, some schizophrenics respond better to high doses of vitamin B_6 and zinc, an essential dietary mineral.

Q. Can vitamin B_{12} improve my memory?

A. It might. A number of studies have found that elderly people with symptoms of senility were deficient in vitamin B_{12}. When they were given supplements of the vitamin, their mental abilities got better. Some other nutrients might also help improve memory, though the effect tends to take several months. Vitamin E and phosphatidyl serine seem to help brain cells function better. So does the herb *Ginkgo biloba*.

Q. What is homocysteine, and why should I be concerned about it?

A. Homocysteine is a byproduct of protein found in the blood. High blood levels of homocysteine damage blood vessel walls and set the stage for cholesterol deposits, ultimately increasing the risk of coronary heart disease. Unlike cholesterol, you will not find homocysteine in foods. Elevated homocysteine levels come about when a person consumes too much protein relative to B vitamins.

A number of B vitamins are involved in breaking down homocysteine or recycling it back to protein. Of these vitamins, folic acid appears to be the most important, but vitamins B_6 and B_{12} are important as well.

New, faster, and relatively inexpensive ways to test for homocysteine levels became available to doctors in 1998. In general, the lower the homocysteine level, the better, and levels of less than 6 micromoles per liter of blood is ideal. Amounts of 10 micromoles per liter of blood used to be considered normal, but this level is increasingly interpreted as risky. The risk increases with the level, and more than 13 micromoles per liter is considered very dangerous. Supplements of 400 mcg of folic acid daily should normalize elevated homocysteine levels. Again, it may be best to take this amount as part of a B-complex supplement.

Q. You recommend individual B vitamins, but you also say I should take a B-complex supplement. Can you clear up the confusion?

A. Individual B vitamins can have a profound and

positive effect on your health. But the eleven B vitamins are part of a closely knit family. If you take large amounts of one B vitamin, it's good to also take a B-complex supplement (or a multivitamin). For example, if you find that vitamin B_1 improves your mood, keep taking it but add a B-complex supplement or a multivitamin. This will make your supplementation even more effective.

Q. When I take B vitamins, my urine turns bright yellow. What's wrong?

A. Nothing is wrong. Vitamin B_2 is naturally yellow, and excess amounts of this vitamin spill into the urine, creating the color. There is absolutely nothing to worry about.

4.

Vitamin C

Vitamin C is abundant in fruits and vegetables, but study after study has found that most people do not eat as many of these foods as they should for good health. Have you eaten your three to five (or as some organizations recommend, five to nine) servings of fruits and vegetables today? Probably not. And for that reason alone, you probably could benefit from vitamin C supplements. Vitamin C can help you resist fatigue and fight infections. It also reduces your risk of cancer, heart disease, and arthritis.

Q. How does vitamin C work?

A. Vitamin C works by enhancing your immune system's ability to fight infections. It increases the activity of white blood cells, T-cells, and antibodies—all of which help kill bacteria and viruses. It also cleans up excess free radicals, which your body produces to fight bacteria and viruses.

Q. Is it true that vitamin C helps prevent, or at least eases, cold and flu symptoms?

A. In 1970, Nobel laureate Linus Pauling, PhD, wrote a book called *Vitamin C and the Common Cold*. In it, he recommends large doses of vitamin C. According to scientific studies published since then, Pauling was pretty much on target. Vitamin C can reduce the symptoms and the length of colds and flus. It cannot prevent them, though. The best prevention is washing your hands after coming into contact with an infected person.

There have been literally dozens of scientific studies that have looked at vitamin C's effects on the common cold. Harri Hemilä, PhD, a researcher at the University of Helsinki, Finland, analyzed these studies as a group. He found that 2 to 6 g (2,000 to 6,000 mg) of vitamin C daily, beginning at the first symptoms of a cold, cut the cold's length and severity by about 30 percent. That means vitamin C can reduce the length of a cold by a couple of days, as well as make its symptoms more tolerable. The minimal effective dose appeared to be 1 g (1,000 mg) daily.

Q. Is vitamin C used to combat very serious infections?

A. For years, Robert Cathcart III, MD, of Los Altos, California, has recommended high doses of vitamin C to patients with very serious infections, including mononucleosis and HIV/AIDS. Cathcart has used extremely high doses—from 25 to 100 g daily—to treat these severe infections.

Q. How do I determine the best dose of vitamin C for me?

A. Most people can benefit from 1,000 to 2,000 mg of vitamin C daily. Even 500 mg daily are better than nothing. If you're willing to take higher dosages, follow Cathcart's concept of adjusting the dose to "bowel tolerance." Cathcart recommends that you increase your vitamin C dose (divided up several times daily) until your stools become loose, and that you then lower your dose slightly.

Cathcart has found that bowel tolerance increases when a person is sick; the sicker a person is, the more vitamin C he or she can tolerate without diarrhea. For example, when you're in good health, you may be able to tolerate only 1 to 3 g of vitamin C over the course of a day. (This will vary from person to person.) If you get a run-of-the-mill cold, your vitamin C tolerance may increase to 10 g per day. If you get a very bad cold, your vitamin C tolerance may increase to 25 g per day. As you start to get better, your vitamin C requirements will decrease. You'll be able to tell this because you'll be more likely to have diarrhea at those high doses. For most people, the ideal dose of vitamin C is just under the amount that causes loose stools and diarrhea. Divide up your dosage so that you take a little vitamin C two to four times a day, instead of all at once. For example, you might try taking 500 mg with breakfast, 500 mg with lunch, 500 mg with dinner, and 500 mg before bed.

Q. Is it important to divide up my daily intake of vitamin C?

A. As stated above, it's best to take a little vitamin C several times daily, or once an hour when you're awake. By taking smaller doses more often, you increase absorption of vitamin C and reduce the likelihood of developing diarrhea.

Q. Do I really need that much vitamin C?

A. Yes. Most animals make their own vitamin C in their bodies, and they make more of it when they're under stress. Based on the amount most animals produce, people would need about 10 to 13 g of vitamin C daily. A genetic defect, which occurred millions of years ago in our evolutionary ancestors, prevents our bodies from producing vitamin C today. So we need to get it from foods or supplements.

Q. I heard that too much vitamin C damages our DNA, the material that makes up our genes. What's the story here?

A. A study published in 1998 found that a dose of 500 mg of vitamin C damaged DNA. But the study was widely criticized by scientists. The results seemed to be caused by contamination during the experiment.

Q. Hasn't vitamin C been recommended for cancer patients?

A. In the 1970s, Ewan Cameron, MD, of Scotland, treated terminal cancer patients with large doses of vitamin C. In general, they lived longer than did patients not given vitamin C, and a small number of them were considered "cured." In addition, over the past ten years, Abram Hoffer, MD, PhD, of Victoria, Canada, has treated terminal cancer patients with large doses of vitamin C combined with other vitamins and minerals. About one-third of his earliest patients, who were judged terminal, are still alive after ten years and are considered by conventional criteria to be cured.

Some types of cancer respond better than others to vitamin C. For example, women with reproductive cancers (such as breast cancer) respond to vitamin therapy much better than people with lung cancer. Hoffer's cancer regimen includes the follow nutrients on a daily basis: 12 g or more of vitamin C; 500 to 3,000 mg of vitamin B_3; 250 mg of vitamin B_6, for some patients; 5 to 10 mg of folic acid; 25 to 50 times the RDA of the other B vitamins; 800 IU of vitamin E, in the "succinate" form; 25,000 to 50,000 IU of the carotenoids; 200 to 600 mcg of selenium; 220 mg of zinc (or 59 mg of zinc citrate); and 300 mg of coenzyme Q_{10}. Doses may vary from patient to patient.

Of course, if you have cancer, it's best to work with a physician instead of treating yourself. If you have already had surgery, chemotherapy, or radiation, these supplements can enhance your immune system so your body does a better job of fighting recurrent cancer.

Q. Can vitamin C help relieve arthritis and rheumatism?

A. It can, though it likely works best in combination with B-complex vitamins. In a recent issue of the French medical journal *Revue Du Rhumatisme*, Jean Léone, MD, of the Robert Debré Teaching Hospital in Reims, describes how two patients who had rheumatism were actually suffering from scurvy. The rheumatism was the presenting symptom. *Scurvy* is a severe vitamin C deficiency disease. Léone patients recovered after he gave them 1,000 mg of vitamin C daily for ten days.

Scurvy is typically characterized by bleeding gums and other types of abnormal bleeding, such as wounds that do not heal. The bleeding is caused by weak capillary walls. (Capillaries are the body's tiniest blood vessels.) In rheumatism and rheumatoid arthritis, weak capillaries leak blood cells into the joints. The immune system responds as if these blood cells were invading bacteria, triggering an inflammatory response.

Supplemental vitamin C strengthens capillary walls, as do antioxidant flavonoids (vitamin-like nutrients found in fruits and vegetables), preventing the leakage of blood vessels and the inflammatory response. Vitamin C is also essential for the body's manufacture of *collagen*, a protein needed to form the soft tissue in bone joints and the skin.

Q. Does vitamin C have any effect on TMJ disease?

A. TMJ disease, or temporomandibular disease, is a type of arthritis that afflicts the joints that connect the jaw to the rest of the head. It can be a painful condition that hinders the chewing of food. Dentists have tended to see TMJ disease as a mechanical problem, which it is. But like arthritic joints, it may be ameliorated by taking antioxidant vitamins.

The research on antioxidants and TMJ disease at this point is only preliminary. Stephen B. Milam, DDS, PhD, and his colleagues at the University of Texas Health Sciences Center, San Antonio, recently wrote about the role of free radicals in amplifying TMJ pain. Because the dental profession has largely ignored antioxidants and other vitamins, Milam cautiously suggested that antioxidants might be of benefit. Remember, vitamin C is an antioxidant. So it is highly likely that it can work to relieve pain due to TMJ.

Q. Why would antioxidants help in TMJ and arthritis?

A. In addition to helping build tissue, antioxidants tend to have an anti-inflammatory effect, and arthritis and TMJ are aggravated by inflammation. Many people take ibuprofen and aspirin to reduce inflammation, but these drugs have undesirable side effects, while antioxidants do not. Antioxidants help regulate the immune system, so they improve your responses to infection and reduce your symptoms. They also calm an over-active immune system, reducing inflammation. Vitamin C is an important anti-inflammatory. Vitamin E also combats inflammation, but its effect is more subtle. Pycnogenol, which is rich in natural nonvitamin antioxidants, is also a powerful anti-inflammatory.

Q. Is it true that vitamin C can prevent cataracts?

A. In a remarkable study directed by Allen Taylor, PhD, of Tufts University, Boston, vitamin C supplements dramatically reduced the risk of developing cataracts. Cataracts involve a clouding of the eye's lens, which impairs vision. They can be caused by excessive exposure to sunlight or by underlying health problems. Diabetics have a high risk of developing cataracts. Keep in mind that cataracts may be a sign of other looming health problems. While cataracts are easily corrected with surgery (in which the lens is removed and replaced by a plastic one), it's always best to avoid surgery. So why not keep up with your vitamin C supplements?

In the study, Taylor found that women who took at least 400 mg of vitamin C supplements daily for more than ten years were about 80-percent likely to develop cataracts. Dietary vitamin C didn't offer this protection. Women who obtained about 130 mg of vitamin C from foods—more than twice the RDA—gained no protection against cataracts.

Q. Can vitamin C help my allergies?

A. Years ago, Robert Cathcart III, MD, became interested in vitamin C because it relieved his hay fever symptoms. During allergic reactions, the body releases a compound called *histamine*, which makes you red and itchy. Vitamin C helps because it has a slight antihistaminic effect, but does not have any of the negative side effects associated with antihistamine drugs. For example, it will not make you drowsy. Vitamin C is also essential for normal immune function, and it likely corrects some of the immune defects involved in allergies.

Q. I have gallbladder problems. Will vitamin C help or harm me?

A. Your gallbladder stores bile, a substance that helps digest fats. An estimated 20 million Americans suffer from gallstones, and the typical person with gallbladder disorders is the overweight, middle-aged woman. One recent study found that vitamin C supplements might reduce the risk of gallbladder disease.

Joel A. Simon, MD, of the University of California, San Francisco, analyzed the health and habits of 2,744 women. He found that women consuming large amounts of vitamin C—particularly through supplements—had a 26-percent lower risk of developing gallbladder disease (of all types) and a 23-percent lower risk of having their gallbladders removed, when compared with women consuming little vitamin C. Vitamin C was especially protective among women who drank alcohol. This subgroup had one-half the risk of developing gallbladder disease and were 62-percent less likely to have their gallbladders removed.

Q. What are the first signs of vitamin C deficiency?

A. The first signs of vitamin C deficiency are tiredness and irritability, according to a recent study by Mark Levine, MD, PhD, of the National Institutes of Health. These are very common symptoms, and there's evidence that many people do not obtain enough vitamin C. More advanced signs of inadequate vitamin C intake are bleeding gums, bruising, sores that take a long time to heal, frequent colds, and extreme fatigue.

5.

Vitamin D

Vitamin D is one of those vitamins that dietitians and nutritionists incorrectly assume most people get enough of. Low vitamin D intake may actually be fairly common. Deficiencies should certainly be remedied, for vitamin D works with calcium, an essential mineral, to help build strong bones and teeth. Thus, it plays an important role in preventing osteoporosis, the thinning of bones that occurs in old age.

Q. I thought calcium was the most important nutrient for healthy bones. What is vitamin D's role?

A. Without vitamin D, calcium cannot be used to build bones. In a study reported in the *New England Journal of Medicine*, Bess Dawson-Hughes, MD, of Tufts University, Boston, gave calcium/vitamin D supplements to one group of participants and dummy pills to the other group. The study involved several hundred elderly men and women. The combination of calcium (500 mg daily) and vitamin D (700 IU daily) increased bone density in the subjects. By the way, vitamin B_{12} and the mineral boron are also important for maintaining healthy bones.

Q. Can vitamin D combat osteoarthritis?

A. In a study, Timothy E. McAlindon, MD, of the Boston University Arthritis Center found that patients were more likely to have osteoarthritis of the knees if they did not consume 400 IU of vitamin D daily. Vitamin D has hormone-like roles in the body, so it probably influences the growth of cells involved in healthy joints. This is yet another way that vitamin D positively affects bone health.

Q. Can vitamin D give me more energy?

A. While vitamin D is not generally considered an "energy nutrient," it does seem to help some people. Konstantinos Ziambaras, MD, and Samuel Dagogo-Jack, MD, writing in the *Western Journal of Medicine*, noted that muscle weakness is associated with vitamin D deficiency. They described two patients with muscle pain and weakness who were deficient in vitamin D. After receiving supplemental vitamin D, their energy levels rose and their muscle pain disappeared.

Q. Don't people get enough vitamin D through food such as fortified milk?

A. Children might, but not all milk is fortified with vitamin D, and many adults don't drink much milk anyway. Your body can actually make its own vitamin D if you spend at least fifteen minutes daily in the sun. But many people with office jobs, or elderly people restricted to home, don't get outside. In the winter, it's more difficult to spend time outdoors, and it's often cloudy.

In a study of 290 patients, Melissa K. Thomas, MD, PhD, of Massachusetts General Hospital, Boston, found that 164 patients over the age of sixty-five were deficient in vitamin D, and 22 percent were severely deficient. But, according to Thomas, even a large number of younger patients who were generally healthy turned out to be deficient in vitamin D. Thomas found that 42 percent of men and women ranging from the late thirties to the late fifties in age were low in vitamin D. So, considering that many individuals are actually vitamin D deficient, it is important to consider supplementation.

Q. What about dosages?

A. Taking 400 to 800 IU of vitamin D daily is safe

for adults. The RDA is 400 IU of daily. Very high doses of vitamin D for extended periods of time can be toxic. Overdosing on vitamin D can cause loss of appetite, nausea, diarrhea, headaches, restlessness, and fatigue. Severe overdosing can result in too much calcium in the blood, which can lead to dangerous calcium deposits in the organs.

6.

Vitamin E

Years ago, doctors dismissed vitamin E as the "sex vitamin" and a "cure in search of a disease." Yet time has been on this amazing vitamin's side. Studies have demonstrated beyond any doubt that vitamin E supplements can reduce your risk of coronary heart disease and stroke. It can slow the progression of Alzheimer's disease and maybe even prevent it. It can even help enhance your immune system. Vitamin E isn't a cure-all, but it does work at a fundamental level in your body, helping it perform the way nature meant it to.

Q. Is vitamin E really good for the heart?

A. In the 1940s, Evan Shute, MD, and his brother Wilfrid Shute, MD, of Canada, pioneered the use of vitamin E supplements in the prevention and treatment of coronary heart disease. Even *Time* magazine wrote about their work in 1946. But at that time, most doctors believed vitamins cured only vitamin-deficiency diseases, not conditions like heart disease. So while the Shutes went on to treat tens of thousands of patients with vitamin E over the years, most doctors felt vitamin E was worthless.

Researchers, meanwhile, conducted basic studies on vitamin E and found it to be not only a powerful antioxidant, but the body's principal fat-soluble antioxidant. In the early 1990s, researchers at Harvard University reported that supplements of vitamin E greatly reduce the risk of heart disease and heart attacks. Then, the actual turning point was most likely a 1996 study published in the British journal *Lancet,* in which vitamin E supplements—400 to 800 IU daily—were found to reduce the incidence of heart attack by 77 percent. Since then, vitamin E has practically become a standard part of mainstream medicine. Many physicians take vitamin E themselves and recommend it to their patients, too.

Q. Will vitamin E help me to attain a healthy heart even if I'm eating a high-fat diet?

A. It will, but obviously you should try to eat better foods. In a study described in the *Journal of the American Medical Association,* Gary D. Plotnick, MD, of the University of Maryland School of Medicine, Baltimore, found that high-fat foods prevent blood vessels from relaxing. Basically, fatty foods trigger a chain of chemical reactions that tense up blood vessels. The long-term effect is to increase blood pressure and the risk of heart disease. When Plotnick gave his subjects (men and women) vitamin E and vitamin C supplements, their blood vessels behaved normally, as if they had eaten low-fat foods.

Q. Will vitamin E do anything for my cholesterol?

A. Vitamin E won't lower your cholesterol level, but it will help to keep cholesterol from damaging your blood vessels, which may be more important. The so-called "bad" form of cholesterol—the low-density lipoproteins (LDLs)—actually is necessary for transporting vitamin E and the carotenoids through the bloodstream. When there is insufficient vitamin E in the LDL cholesterol, it is prone to oxidation—that is, to free radical damage. This oxidized LDL cholesterol infiltrates blood vessel walls much more than normal, nonoxidized LDL cholesterol. In studies involving human subjects, Ishwarlal Jialal, MD, of the University of Texas Southwestern Medical Center, Dallas, found that vitamin E supplements protect LDLs from oxida-

tion, thus preventing LDL deposits in blood vessels
and reducing the risk of coronary heart disease.

Q. I'm heading in for heart surgery. Is it too late to take vitamin E?

A. It's never too late, though you should discuss
vitamin E with your heart doctor. There is substantial
research showing that vitamin E and other antioxidant vitamins can reduce the risk of complications
from heart surgery. This is important because heart
surgery is a major stress, and about 3 percent of people undergoing bypass surgery do not survive.

During bypass surgery, blood flow is stopped so
doctors can graft new arteries. When blood flow is
replenished, large numbers of free radicals are gen-
erated, and these radicals can damage the heart. For
this reason, some heart surgeons give their patients
vitamin E supplements before surgery. Vitamin C
and coenzyme Q_{10} may also be helpful here.

In one study, Howard N. Hodis, MD, of the
University of Southern California School of Medicine, Los Angles, found that patients taking 100 to 450
IU of vitamin E developed smaller heart lesions (cholesterol deposits) than patients not taking the vitamin.
All of Hodis' subjects had already had bypass surgery. So vitamin E seems to help at every stage of cardiovascular disease.

Q. Breast cancer runs in my family. Would vitamin E help reduce my risk?

A. Vitamin E may very well reduce your risk of breast cancer. Japanese researchers at the Okayama University Medical School conducted a very interesting study along these lines. Apparently, some people have a genetic defect that interferes with their body's production of *catalase*, an antioxidant enzyme. As many as 6 million Americans may have this genetic defect. Without sufficient catalase, cells have trouble neutralizing free radicals, which go on to damage the cells and increase the risk of cancer. So the researchers studied mice that did not produce enough catalase. They found that these catalase-deficient mice were more likely to develop breast cancers. But when the researchers added vitamin E to the diets, the mice were far less likely to develop breast cancer.

The question comes up as to whether vitamin E would have the same benefit in people. According to the researchers, who published their findings in the *Japanese Journal of Cancer Research*, "vitamin E intrinsically has a protective effect against the development of mammary tumor, and this may apply . . . to humans."

Q. Would vitamin E cause any problems in a diabetic?

A. Every diabetic taking insulin or hypoglycemic drugs should start taking vitamins in small amounts and gradually increase the doses, unless his or her physician advises otherwise. Because most vitamins are involved in converting blood sugar (glucose) to energy, vitamins may speed up this process and lower glucose levels quickly. So exercise caution at first.

The good news is that all diabetics can benefit from vitamin supplementation. You see, glucose generates large numbers of free radicals, and this gets out of hand in diabetics because they have high glucose levels. These free radicals oxidize cholesterol and damage blood vessel walls. This is one reason why diabetics have an above-average risk of developing cardiovascular diseases. Vitamin E and alpha-lipoic acid, a vitamin-like antioxidant, help control these excess free radicals and reduce the damage. Alpha-lipoic acid (300 to 600 mg daily, for diabetics) may lower glucose levels by 10 to 30 percent, and the glucose levels also stabilize, which is better for controlling diabetes. Other vitamins, such as vitamin C and the B-complex, help control diabetes and diabetic complications as well.

Q. Can vitamin E cure Alzheimer's disease?

A. "Cure" is too strong of a term, but it can certainly slow the progression of this devastating disease. Mary Sano, PhD, of Columbia University's College of Physicians and Surgeons, New York, and her colleagues gave severe Alzheimer's patients 2,000 IU of vitamin E (a very large dose!), selegiline (a drug used to treat Parkinson's disease), a combination of the two, or a placebo daily for two years. Vitamin E delayed the progression of end-stage Alzheimer's disease by eight months, compared with the placebo. Selegiline worked almost as well, but not quite. The combination helped a little, but not as much as either vitamin E or selegiline alone. After Sano's study was published in the *New England Journal of Medicine*, the American Psychiatric Association recommended that Alzheimer's patients receive vitamin E. Sano is planning another study to determine whether taking high doses of vitamin E might help early-stage Alzheimer's patients.

Q. Why would vitamin E help combat Alzheimer's disease?

A. Vitamin E is essential for the normal functioning of cell membranes, or cell walls. These cell membranes have doors that allow vitamins and other nutrients to come in and waste products to go out. With age, the membranes harden. Vitamin E seems to keep them more supple. In addition, vitamin E limits free radical damage to brain cells. This is important because high levels of free radicals are thought to be a major cause of Alzheimer's disease.

Q. What about vitamin E and infection?

A. Although most people don't see vitamin E as an immune booster, several studies show that it can enhance resistance to infection. This is particularly important for older folks, because the immune system declines with age. In a study at Tufts University, Boston, researchers found that 200 IU of vitamin E daily improved immune responsiveness by 65 percent. This means the immune system would be more likely to respond to infection during a bacterial attack. The researchers also noted that people taking vitamin E had 30-percent fewer infections. Other studies have found that vitamin E (as well as selenium) can prevent dangerous mutations in the coxsackie virus, which infects some 20 million Americans a year with sore throats and cold-like symptoms.

Q. Some of my friends snicker and call vitamin E the "sex vitamin." Will it make me perform better?

A. When vitamin E was discovered in 1922, it was called the "fertility vitamin" because rodents deficient in vitamin E became sterile. Being infertile, of course, is different from being impotent. Still, people started referring to vitamin E as the "sex vitamin." Actually, vitamin E can help some men with impotency, though the improvement won't occur overnight. The reason is that most cases of impotence are related to cardiovascular disease. In impotency, the blood vessels of the penis become as damaged as those of the heart. So anything that improves cardiovascular disease—such as vitamin E—may also help in impotency.

Vitamin E probably helps in impotency for another reason. It improves blood flow to tissues—all tissues, including those in the penis. Every condition improves with better blood flow. However, if you are impotent because of psychological reasons, such as the bedroom version of stage fright, vitamin E probably won't help.

Q. Can vitamin E help us conceive and become parents?

A. Several studies published in *Fertility and Sterility* have reported that infertile men have high levels of free radicals and low levels of antioxidants in their semen. For this reason, many urologists recommend vitamin E and other antioxidants to such men. It takes at least three months for vitamins to have an effect, mainly because it takes that long for sperm to mature. In general, both members of an infertile couple should take supplemental vitamin E and a high-potency multivitamin for several months before trying to conceive.

Q. Sometimes when I exercise, I really feel wiped out. Can vitamin E reduce this fatigue?

A. According to Lester Packer, PhD, a researcher at the University of California, Berkeley, and one of the foremost authorities on antioxidants, vitamin E can probably reduce exercise-induced fatigue. Quicker recovery from fatigue will improve general exercise performance.

Your body's cells produce free radicals as a

byproduct of normal activities. When you exercise, you speed up the process and generate more free radicals. So, ironically, excessive exercise is bad. The solution, though, is not to become a couch potato; it's to take vitamin E and other antioxidants. These vitamins prevent DNA (genetic) damage and oxidation of cell fats caused by over-exercise.

Q. What's the typical dose of vitamin E?

A. Most experts seem to have settled on 400 IU of vitamin E daily as the healthy dose. Some studies have shown that levels as low as 100 IU provide some benefit and that higher doses—800 IU to 1,200 IU—are safe, though probably unnecessary. Natural vitamin E is preferable to the synthetic form.

Q. Can I get this amount of vitamin E through my diet?

A. No. In an editorial in the journal *Geriatrics*, Robert N. Butler, MD, states that you would have to eat 1,000 almonds to get 400 IU of vitamin E—and all of those almonds would contain 8,000 calories and more than a pound of fat.

Our vitamin E requirements are very high, in part, because we eat large quantities of refined oils (in salad dressings, french fries, and many other foods). These oils are very prone to oxidation, and vitamin E protects against their oxidation. So the more fats you eat through refined oils, the higher your vitamin E needs.

Q. Is there a difference between natural and synthetic vitamin E?

A. There is a big difference. Synthetic vitamin E contains eight components called *stereoisomers*. Only one of these is the same as that found in natural vitamin E. Over the years, studies found that milligram for milligram, natural vitamin E was about 36-percent more biologically active than the synthetic form. The IU, or international unit, standard was developed to equalize this difference. But natural vitamin E is still superior to the synthetic.

A recent study by Graham W. Burton, PhD, of Canada's National Research Council, found that natural vitamin E was absorbed twice as efficiently as the synthetic. In human test subjects, natural vitamin E levels rose twice as high as the synthetic. This means that, even using the current IU standard, natural vitamin E is 66-percent better absorbed than the synthetic. Basically, you get more for your money by purchasing natural vitamin E.

Q. So, how do I tell the difference between natural and synthetic vitamin E?

A. Look at the fine print on the label. Synthetic vitamin E will be identified by its chemical name, "dl-alpha tocopherol" or "dl-alpha tocopheryl acetate." It's the "dl" you have to watch out for. In contrast, natural vitamin E comes as "d-alpha tocopherol," "d-alpha tocopheryl acetate," or "d-alpha tocopheryl succinate." These are different vitamin E compounds, but the key here is the "d," which indicates that the substance is the natural form. Most natural vitamin E, by the way, comes from soybeans.

7.

Vitamin K

Many people have never heard of vitamin K. Yet this vitamin plays important roles in the health of the bloodstream and in bone formation. Like many other vitamins, it appears that most people may not be obtaining enough of it through diet.

Q. What is vitamin K?

A. Vitamin K, also called phylloquinone, is a fat-soluble vitamin closely related to coenzyme Q_{10}. Without Vitamin K, you would bleed to death from the slightest scratch. It is needed to help blood-platelet cells clot after a cut or incision. It is also essential for brain development. According to M. J. Shearer, PhD, of St. Thomas' Hospital, London, babies deficient in this vitamin during the first six months of their lives risk permanent brain damage or death.

Q. What does vitamin K have to do with bone formation?

A. The most recent research has emphasized the role of vitamin K in the formation of bone. In other words, healthy bones depend on more than just calcium and vitamin D. To explain, *osteocalcin* is one of the proteins involved in bone development. To build bone, osteocalcin must be loaded by chemical structures known as carboxyl groups. Your body uses vitamin K to help attach these carboxyl groups to osteocalcin. In a study of nine healthy women at Tufts University, Boston, James A. Sadlowski, PhD, found that vitamin K supplements increase the attachment of carboxyl groups to osteocalcin, setting the stage for bone formation.

Q. How much vitamin K do I need to achieve this bone-building effect?

A. Sadlowski's study used 420 mcg of vitamin K daily, which is about four times the RDA. According to an article in the *Journal of Nutrition*, levels of vitamin K in most foods are pretty low. One of the best dietary sources is green leafy vegetables. However, absorption of vitamin K from foods is poor, so supplementing may be beneficial. If you take a multivitamin, make sure there's some vitamin K in it.

8.

Vitamin-Like Nutrients

By definition, vitamins are essential dietary nutrients. Then there are many *vitamin-like* nutrients, including coenzyme Q_{10} (CoQ_{10}), carnitine, alpha-lipoic acid, and N-acetylcysteine. These substances function in ways similar to vitamins. They are not considered true vitamins because your body is capable of producing them, or because obtaining them from dietary sources has not yet been deemed essential for health. Nonetheless, they are highly beneficial nutrients. Unfortunately, some people do not produce adequate amounts of them. For this reason, either foods high in these nutrients or supplements that include them help promote good health.

Q. What is coenzyme Q_{10}, or CoQ_{10}?

A. Coenzyme Q_{10} plays a key role in how the body's cells "burn" food into energy. Its chemical name is ubiquinone—the "ubi" term refers to it being ubiquitous, or existing throughout nature. So important is CoQ_{10} that it was the basis of the 1978 Nobel prize in chemistry. After sugar and fat are broken down to their most basic molecules, submolecular particles called electrons and protons carry energy from one part of the cell to another. CoQ_{10} functions like a shuttle bus, moving these electrons and protons through two key energy-producing steps.

Q. How does CoQ_{10} help the heart?

A. The heart is probably the most energetic organ in the body. As such, it is very dependent on energy-converting compounds, such as CoQ_{10}. In fact, scientists isolated the first CoQ_{10} from the hearts of cows. In the 1970s, Japanese and American physicians began giving CoQ_{10} to patients with cardiomyopathy (an enlarged but weak heart) and heart failure. These types of heart disease are caused by a lack of heart energy, rather than by too much cholesterol. The supplemental CoQ_{10} not only strengthened but also reduced the abnormally large size of the hearts of these patients—a sign of more efficient heart function.

Severe cardiomyopathy and heart failure are often surgically remedied through heart transplants, but such surgeries are expensive. In addition, there are only about 2,000 hearts available per year for transplants, whereas there are about 2 million Americans with these severe heart diseases. CoQ_{10} is an effective—and natural—way of correcting cardiomyopathy and heart failure. In fact, many people scheduled for heart transplants have been able to avoid surgery because of CoQ_{10}. While the dosage varies from patient to patient, most seem to benefit from 300 to 400 mg daily.

There's only one cautionary note. While CoQ_{10} is safe, care should be taken if you are taking heart-stimulating drugs, such as digitalis. The combination could overstimulate the heart. If you are taking such medication, work with your physician to adjust the dosage of the drug, while increasing your CoQ_{10} intake.

Q. What about CoQ_{10} and cancer?

A. Knud Lockwood, MD, of Copenhagen, Denmark, has assigned CoQ_{10} supplementation of 390 mg daily to prevent the recurrence of breast cancer in his patients. Lockwood had treated breast cancer conventionally for thirty-five years. When he started giving CoQ_{10} to patients, their new breast cancers receded. Lockwood reported that he had never before seen such remissions.

CoQ$_{10}$ is not directly an anti-tumor compound. It appears to enhance the functioning of the immune system, perhaps by increasing the energy levels of immune cells and enabling them to do a better job when fighting cancers. Because of this general immune-enhancing effect, CoQ$_{10}$ also increases resistance to infections.

Q. Will CoQ$_{10}$ improve my energy levels?

A. Many people say that CoQ$_{10}$ does increase your energy level. It's hard to tell, without testing, whether a person's CoQ$_{10}$ levels are normal or below normal. Taking 30 to 100 mg daily may relieve fatigue in otherwise healthy patients. In a small study, Langsjoen found that CoQ$_{10}$ supplements increased energy levels in people in their eighties. So it seems promising that this vitamin-like nutrient will give you more "get-up-and-go."

Q. What is alpha-lipoic acid, and how does it help diabetics?

A. Alpha-lipoic acid—or lipoic acid, for short—also helps cells to convert food to energy by improving the breakdown of sugar. Lipoic acid is so efficient at this that it has been used for years in Germany as a "drug" for diabetes. Originally, alpha-lipoic acid was used to treat diabetic polyneuropathy, a group of nerve disorders in diabetics. These disorders can result in pain or numbness. The numbness is dangerous because a diabetic with neuropathy (nerve disease) of the foot may not know, for example, that he has injured his foot. As a result, infection and gangrene, to which diabetics are especially vulnerable, may set in. Diabetic patients generally benefit from 200 mg of lipoic acid, taken three times daily (totaling 600 mg daily).

Q. Can alpha-lipoic acid help diabetics in other ways?

A. Because lipoic acid improves the breakdown of sugar, it helps lower and stabilize blood sugar (glucose) levels. Diabetics need to be aware of this effect, so that they can be prepared to adjust the levels of insulin or hypoglycemic drugs that they may be taking. On average, a daily intake of 600 mg of lipoic acid lowers glucose levels by 10 to 20 percent.

According to Lester Packer, PhD, of the University of California, Berkeley, lipoic acid is a very powerful antioxidant. It works as an antioxidant by itself, in its dihydrolipoic acid form (which the body makes from lipoic acid), and by helping to regenerate other antioxidants, such as vitamins C and E. High levels of glucose "auto-oxidize" in the body. In other words, the high glucose levels start a chain reaction that generates large numbers of free radicals. Researchers believe that many of the complications of diabetes, including an above-average risk of heart disease, are due, in part, to these excess free radicals. Lipoic acid quenches many of these free radicals and helps other antioxidants work harder to do the same. And by lowering glucose levels, it also reduces the number of free radicals produced.

Q. What is carnitine, and how does it work?

A. Carnitine is a component of protein that helps the body's cells burn fats. Unburned fats are stored as triglycerides, a type of fat that is (like cholesterol) associated with increased risk of heart disease. So carnitine works against this accumulation of triglycerides and the subsequent threat of cardiovascular disease.

Carnitine supplements have been helpful to many people with chronic fatigue syndrome (CSF). In a study at the Mercy Hospital and Medical Center, Chicago, physicians found that CFS patients taking 3 g of carnitine daily had significant improvements in energy levels after eight weeks.

Q. Is acetyl-L-carnitine related to carnitine?

A. Acetyl-L-carnitine is a slightly different form of the same nutrient. The "acetyl" prefix comes from the fact that acetyl-L-carnitine has an "acetyl group" attached to the carnitine molecule. An acetyl group consists of chemicals similar to those found in acetic acid, or common vinegar.

Several studies have found that acetyl-L-carnitine supplements can slow the progression of Alzheimer's disease. In one study, reported in the journal *Neurology*, Leon J. Thal, MD, of the University of California, San Diego, reported that patients taking acetyl-L-carnitine had a slower progression of the disease, compared with patients taking dummy pills.

Q. Do carnitine and acetyl-L-carnitine have an anti-aging effect?

A. There is some research, yet unpublished, showing that acetyl-L-carnitine has an anti-aging effect in laboratory animals. The studies appear scientifically sound. Also, carnitine helps maintain cell levels of *cardiolipin*, a substance needed to maintain cell-membrane flexibility. Cell membranes act like the walls and doors of cells. As long as they are flexible, they allow important nutrients into cells, while letting waste products out. Carnitine, therefore, keeps the cells functioning youthfully, which, in turn, allows our bodies to function youthfully.

Q. What is N-acetylcysteine and what is it known to do?

A. Cysteine is an amino acid, or a protein component, found in foods. N-acetylcysteine (like acetyl-L-carnitine) contains an acetyl group. It works largely by increasing the body's production of *glutathione*, a very powerful antioxidant.

A recent study found that N-acetylcysteine supplements can greatly reduce flu and flu-like symptoms. In the study, Italian physicians gave 262 elderly people either 1,200 mg of N-acetylcysteine or a placebo daily for six months, overlapping the winter cold and flu season. Of the subjects who had laboratory-confirmed flus, only 25 percent of those taking N-acetylcysteine developed symptoms, compared with 79 percent of those taking inert placeboes. Among people with more general flu-like symptoms, N-acetylcysteine greatly reduced the severity of symptoms. N-acetylcysteine may be one of the most remarkable flu and cold "medicines" ever discovered.

N-acetylcysteine also helps you to resist disease and the aging process. Most serious diseases are associated with decreased glutathione levels. Even the aging process is associated with low glutathione levels. N-acetylcysteine boosts these levels.

In a study of AIDS patients, Stanford University researchers found that N-acetylcysteine boosted their sagging glutathione and increased their life expectancy. The researchers offered AIDS patients 3,200 to 8,000 mg of N-acetylcysteine daily. Those who took N-acetylcysteine generally lived twice as long as those who declined to take the supplement.

9.

Shopping for and Taking Vitamins

There's no doubt that vitamin supplements are good for your health. But working your way through all of the available supplements, their effects, and their dosages can be confusing. Which ones should you take, and how much of each? Should you take tablets or capsules, natural or synthetic vitamins? This chapter answers some of the questions about buying and using vitamin supplements.

Q. Sometimes I feel like different vitamins do the same things in the body. Why can't I take just one vitamin?

A. All of the vitamins are essential nutrients, and each one of them performs myriad functions in the body. For example, vitamin C, vitamin E, and folic acid reduce the risk of coronary heart disease. But they protect the heart and blood vessels in different ways. Similarly, vitamin C and the B vitamins can ease arthritis, but they do so in different ways.

Given the choice, would you build a house with a strong frame or a weak frame? A weak frame might hold up your walls and roof, but only until a strong wind blows it down. A strong frame would hold up your house in a severe storm. Vitamins are similar. You can certainly improve your health by taking vitamin C supplements, but you could improve it even more by adding vitamin E supplements. The most sensible approach is to take all of the vitamins. If it's a hassle for you to take pills, stick with one high-potency, multivitamin supplement.

Q. Okay, I'm convinced of the benefits of vitamins. How do I start supplementing?

A. Sometimes looking at all the different bottles of vitamins on the shelf can be a little overwhelming. It helps to set some clear objectives. In other words, think about why you want to take a particular supplement. For example, if you're in your twenties, eat a reasonably good diet, and are in good health, your objective might be "dietary insurance." In this case, you could simply take a high-potency multivitamin supplement (which contains all the vitamins). On the other hand, if you're in your thirties or forties and face a lot of stress at home or at work, "stress management" might be an objective. For this goal, you'd probably do well taking a high-potency B-complex supplement as well.

Reducing the risk of disease is a very clear objective. If people in your family have a high risk of developing heart disease or cancer, it's probably wise to start supplementing before the first signs of trouble. Vitamin E would probably be the most important vitamin, along with a multivitamin.

If you have specific health problems, such as high blood pressure, hardening of the arteries, premenstrual syndrome (PMS), or osteoporosis, taking high doses of specific supplements may be in order. For example, the B-vitamin complex can often ease PMS.

By starting with some specific objectives, you've got something to measure your improvement against.

Q. What are mg, mcg, g, and IU?

A. These are units of weight in which vitamins are typically measured. Actually, they are abbreviations for the units of weight. The actual terms are as follows: g stands for grams; mg stands for milligrams; mcg stands for micrograms; and IU stands for international units.

To put these weights into perspective, there are about 454 g in a pound; 1,000 mg in a gram; and

1,000 mcg in a milligram. We're talking about very small quantities, compared with the amounts of nutrients you get in a hamburger patty or a few slices of bread. For example, 400 mcg of folic acid is equivalent to about one seventy-thousandth (1/70,000) of an ounce—a very small quantity, but very important nonetheless. International units (IU), which are a way of measuring vitamins A, D, and E, do not consistently correspond to milligrams.

Q. In general, for well-being and prevention, how much of each vitamin should I take?

A. Specific recommendations vary, but general, safe dosages are provided below. To obtain these amounts, you may have to take more than one tablet or capsule daily. These dosages are for adults.

Vitamin	Daily Dosages
Biotin	30–50 mcg
Choline	250 mg
Folic acid	400 mg
Inositol	250 mg
PABA	30–50 mg

Vitamin	Daily Dosages
Pantothenic acid	25–100 mg
Vitamin A and/or beta-carotene	5,000 IU 15 mg or 25,000 IU
Vitamin B_1 (thiamine)	10–15 mg
Vitamin B_{12}	10–100 mg
Vitamin B_2 (riboflavin)	10–25 mg
Vitamin B_3 (niacinamide)	100–200 mg
Vitamin B_6 (pyridoxine)	10–20 mg
Vitamin C	1,000–4,000 mg
Vitamin E	400 IU
Vitamin K	100 mcg

Tailoring vitamin supplements for children can be trickier because they weigh less. For general supplementation, one or two times the children's RDA (which is set lower than the adult RDA) should be completely safe. But, stick with RDA levels of vitamin A and D for children to avoid an overdose, unless you're getting advice suggesting otherwise from a physician.

Q. Is supplementation safe during pregnancy?

A. Supplementation is *necessary* during pregnancy. If you're already taking a high-potency multivita-

min—one that contains the dosages just described—
you're fine. If you're not, start taking either a multivitamin or a prenatal supplement. The reason is that
vitamins are essential for the normal development of
your fetus. For example, if the fetus does not have
adequate folic acid through its mother's diet by the
sixteenth week of pregnancy, it's neural tube (spine)
will not seal, and the result will be a serious birth
defect such as spina bifida.

A study described in the *Journal of the National
Cancer Institute* found that women who took vitamins while pregnant were less likely to have children with brain tumors. These are compelling reasons to take vitamins before and during pregnancy.
Of course, it's also important not to smoke or drink
alcohol and to eat a balanced diet during pregnancy. Also, keep in mind that it's best to start taking a
vitamin supplement before you become pregnant.

Q. Should I take supplements with food? And at what time of day?

A. Vitamins are components of food, so, in general, they are best taken with food. It's also a good
idea to take your vitamins with breakfast, so that
your body has them to use when you're most active.
Another reason to take your vitamins in the morn-
ing is that they tend to have a stimulatory effect.

Many vitamins are involved in the production of energy. Furthermore, if you take your vitamins before going to bed, you may have a restless night. For example, vitamin B_6 will increase the vividness of your dreams.

Sometimes vitamin labels recommend taking supplements two or three times a day, one with each meal. In such cases, follow the directions on the label. And if you're taking large amounts of a single vitamin, such as several tablets of vitamin C, it's best to divide up the dose over the course of a day. Splitting up the dose improves the efficiency of absorption and, therefore, less of your intake is excreted. (You don't have to take vitamin C with food because it's water-soluble and easily absorbed. Dividing up the dose will also reduce the likelihood of loose bowels from taking too much at one time.)

Q. Is there a difference between natural and synthetic vitamins?

A. It depends on the vitamin. Most vitamin supplements are synthetic duplicates of natural vitamins and are identical in all respects. But there is a big difference between natural and synthetic vitamin E. The same goes for beta-carotene. In both cases, the natural form is superior to the synthetic.

Graham Burton, PhD, a researcher at the National

Research Council of Canada, Ottawa, has shown the human body assimilates the natural form of vitamin E twice as efficiently as the synthetic. Essentially, as Burton says, you get "more bang for your buck." You can tell the difference by looking at the fine print on supplement bottles: "d-alpha tocopherol" indicates natural, and "dl-alpha tocopherol" indicates synthetic. Tocopherol (also spelled tocopheryl) is the chemical name for vitamin E.

Most sources of natural beta-carotene supplements are derived from the *Dunaliella salina* algae. (This should also be listed on the label.) Natural beta-carotene consists of two forms that chemists call isomers. The synthetic supplements contain only one of these forms.

You don't need to concern yourself with this issue when it comes to vitamins C, B, A, D, and K. Vitamin C is produced from corn sugar (dextrose), and the B vitamins are produced through bacterial fermentation, basically by cultivating bacteria that produce large amounts of B vitamins. Vitamins A, D, and K come from both natural and synthetic sources, but the differences are not significant.

Q. What are excipients, and are they safe?

A. If you read labels closely, you've probably noticed a lot of nonvitamin substances listed as ingredients. All tablets and capsules contain excipients, which are nonnutritive compounds. They are added to improve the consistency of vitamin supplements during manufacture.

Before vitamins are pressed into tablets or poured into capsules, they are in powder form and thoroughly mixed in vats. Some excipients, such as lubricants, promote consistent mixing. Thus, you get the same amount of a vitamin in every tablet or capsule. Others, such as cellulose, add bulk so that the vitamins can be pressed into tablets. Cellulose also absorbs water, which helps the tablet to swell and break apart in your digestive tract.

All excipients are approved for use by the Food and Drug Administration and are safe. Some people, however, have reactions to certain excipients, such as lactose (milk sugar). If you find this happening to you, switch to a different product. Also, if you're allergic to milk or are lactose intolerant, it might be best to completely avoid supplements containing lactose. Read labels carefully.

Q. How do I choose between a tablet and a capsule?

A. Each form has some advantages and disadvantages. Choosing one over another depends on a variety of factors, including availability, cost, ease of swallowing, and the number of excipients you're willing to ingest.

Most supplements are sold in tablet form. They're less expensive to make than capsules. But capsules are easier to swallow than tablets, particularly when compared with large tablets. Furthermore, sometimes tablets pass through the gut without breaking down. If this happens to you consistently, switch to a capsule. You might also consider taking betaine-hydrochloride or another type of digestive aid to improve your stomach acid.

Some supplements, such as vitamin B_{12}, come in sublingual tablets. These are meant to dissolve under the tongue, much the way nitroglycerin (a heart medication) is taken. A network of blood vessels under the tongue instantly absorbs vitamins and drugs. You'll also find some vitamins in liquid form. Because vitamins generally don't taste very good, these products tend to contain a lot of sugar to mask the taste.

Q. What about time-release vitamins that break down slowly?

A. Generally, when you take a vitamin, it is absorbed into the bloodstream. Blood levels of the vitamin increase for several hours, then drop, and the excess is excreted. The idea behind time-release supplements is that they maintain steadier levels in the blood and, therefore, less is excreted. The disadvantage is the cost of time-release supplements. Some are twice as expensive as regular vitamin supplements. If you are concerned with maintaining more consistent blood levels of your vitamins for a longer period of time, a less expensive approach would be to divide up your vitamins into smaller doses and to take a little with breakfast, lunch, and dinner, instead of all at once.

Q. Should I take a break from taking vitamin supplements, just to give my body a rest?

A. Would you take a break from eating to give your body a rest? No. The same is true with vitamin supplements. If you're taking only a multivitamin, it probably won't matter if you miss a day here or there. But there's no need to intentionally halt your supplementation. And once you start taking vitamins, you'll probably feel so much better that you won't want to stop.

Q. I don't like taking a lot of pills. If I took just one supplement, what should it be?

A. A multivitamin supplement is probably the best choice for you. Most contain all of the vitamins, but there is a great variation in dosage. Because the RDA suggests a conservative amount, look for a supplement that provides at least four times the RDA for the B vitamins, vitamin C, and vitamin E. (Stick with RDA levels for vitamins A and D.)

Q. How do I know if a specific supplement is working?

A. If you're taking a specific supplement to treat a condition—such as B vitamins to treat arthritis—you should see some benefits within about thirty days, assuming you're taking enough. If you don't see an improvement after thirty days, stop taking the supplement. It's possible that your improvement was very subtle and you won't notice it until you stop. Or maybe you would benefit from a different vitamin.

It's a little harder to assess the effects of vitamins if you're in good health and trying to reduce your long-term risk of disease. "That's where the research comes in," says Elson M. Haas, MD, of San Rafael, California. "You're not going to notice that you have fewer free radicals."

The benefits of vitamin supplements will become clearer the longer you take them. You'll find that you'll generally be in better health than people your age who don't take vitamins. "When patients with a variety of maladies start a supplement program, they tend to feel better," Haas adds. "Their friends ask what they're doing. This is very different from drug therapy which tends to produce a lot of unwanted side effects."

Q. What are the limitations of vitamin supplements?

A. This one's easy. Supplements are exactly what the name says—supplements to, not replacements for, good nutrition. They provide dietary insurance, they can compensate somewhat for some subtle biological defects, and they can prevent and treat many diseases. But they won't protect you from a fundamentally bad diet. Eat well, and take your supplements.

Conclusion

When the first vitamins were discovered in 1911, they were understood to be cures only for serious vitamin-deficiency diseases, such as scurvy (hemorrhaging) and beriberi (paralysis). At that time, no one imagined how important vitamins were to overall health, and no one foresaw that vitamins could help reduce the risk of serious diseases, including heart disease and cancer.

In recent years, vitamin research has entered a scientific renaissance. Researchers and increasing numbers of physicians recognize that vitamins play essential roles in maintaining normal health and in helping us resist disease and the aging process itself. At the same time, it's becoming painfully clear that the modern diet of fast foods and the eating habits that come along with our high-pressure, hurried schedules prevent us from getting sufficient amounts of all of the vitamins from foods. This is where vitamin supplements can help. To some extent, they can make up for a bad diet. But their

benefits go far beyond this. Vitamins can help keep
your body functioning optimally. They are agents of
prevention, offering us greater quality and quantity
of life. And that is, fundamentally, what most of us
strive for—a long life, free of disease.

Glossary

Antioxidant. A substance that limits damage from free radicals by donating an electron. Antioxidant nutrients can reduce the risk of heart disease and cancer. Two examples are vitamin C and vitamin E. (*See also* Free radical.)

Enzyme. A catalyst that promotes a biochemical reaction. Vitamins often function as co-enzymes, meaning they work with other enzymes.

Excipient. A non-nutritive ingredient used to manufacture tablets and capsules.

Free radical. An unpaired electron produced by the body or by pollutants. Free radicals are regarded as an underlying cause of aging, heart disease, and cancer. (*See also* Antioxidant.)

Gram (g). A unit of weight. One pound equals 454 grams.

International unit (IU). A unit of weight, usually used for fat-soluble vitamins. For example, 1.49 IU and 1 mg are the same amount of natural vitamin E.

Megavitamin. A term often used to describe high doses of vitamins, such as those above the Recommended Dietary Allowance.

Mineral. An element, such as calcium, essential for health and life.

Microgram (mcg). A unit of weight. A microgram is one-millionth of a gram, or one-thousandth of a milligram.

Milligram (mg). A unit of weight. A milligram is one-thousandth of a gram.

Oil-soluble vitamin. A vitamin that dissolves only in oil. Vitamins A, D, E, and coenzyme Q_{10} are oil soluble and are, therefore, best consumed with oil. The body stores oil-soluble vitamins. (*See also* Water-soluble vitamin.)

Orthomolecular. Literally means "to straighten molecules." Coined by Nobel laureate Linus Pauling, the term refers to the use of natural substances to restore balance to the body's molecules and, thus, health.

Time-release. A term used to describe a vitamin manufactured for the slow release of its ingredient. (Conventional tablets are supposed to disintegrate after forty-five minutes in the digestive tract. Capsules dissolve within a few minutes.)

Vitamin. A micronutrient that is essential for life and health. The body makes some vitamins, but most must be obtained from food or supplements.

Water-soluble vitamin. A vitamin that dissolves in water. Examples are vitamin C and the B complex. Water-soluble vitamins are excreted in about a day or so, and must be replenished. (*See also* Oil-soluble vitamin.)

References

The information in this book is drawn from several hundred scientific references. These are some of those references.

Burton GW, Traber MG, Acuff RV, et al., "Human plasma and tissue a-tocopherol concentrations in response to supplementation with deuterated natural and synthetic vitamin E," *American Journal of Clinical Nutrition* 67 (1998): 669–684.

Cathcart RF, "Vitamin C, titrating to bowel tolerance, anascorbemia, and acute induced scurvy," *Medical Hypotheses* 7 (1981): 1359–1376.

De Flora S, Grassi C, Carati L, "Attenuation of influenza-like symptomology and improvement of cell-mediated immunity with long-term N-acetyl-cysteine treatment," *European Respiratory Journal* 10 (1997): 1535–1541.

Eberlein-König B, Placzek M, and Pryzybilla B, "Protective effect against sunburn of combined systemic ascorbic acid (vitamin C) and d-a-tocopherol (vitamin E)," *Journal of the American Academy of Dermatology* 38 (1998): 45–48.

Heinonen OP, Albanes D, Virtano J, et al., "Prostate cancer and supplementation with a-tocopherol; and b-carotene: incidence and mortality in a controlled trial," *Journal of the National Cancer Institute* 90 (1998): 440–446.

Jacques PF, Taylor A, Hankinson SF, et al., "Long-term vitamin C supplement use and prevalence of early age-related lens opacities," *American Journal of Clinical Nutrition* 66 (1997): 911–916.

Keniston RC, Nathan PA, Leklem JE, et al., "Vitamin B_6, vitamin C, and carpal tunnel syndrome," *Journal of Occupational and Environmental Medicine* 39 (1997): 949–959.

Kodama H, Yamaguchi R, Fukuda J, et al., "Increased oxidative deoxyribonucleic acid damage in the spermatozoa of infertile male patients," *Fertility and Sterility* 68 (1997): 519–524.

Léone J, Delhinger V, Maes D, et al., *Revue Du Rhumatisme* (English edition) 64 (1997): 428–431.

Lin Y, Burri BJ, Neidlinger TR, et al., "Estimating the concentration of b-carotene required for maximal protection of low-density lipoproteins in women," *American Journal of Clinical Nutrition* 67 (1998): 837–845.

Milam SB, Zardeneta G, Schmitz JP, "Oxidative stress and degenerative temporomandibular joint disease: a proposed hypothesis," *Journal of Oral and Maxillofacial Surgery* 56 (1998): 214–222.

Packer L, "Oxidants, antioxidant nutrients and the athlete," *Journal of Sports Sciences* 15 (1997): 353–363.

Plotnick GD, Corretti MC, Vogel RA, "Effect of antioxidant vitamins on the transient impairment of endothelium-dependent brachial artery vasoactivity following a single high-fat meal," *JAMA* 278 (1997): 1682–1686.

Pool-Zobel BL, Bub A, Muller H, et al., "Consumption of vegetables reduces genetic damage in humans: first results of a human intervention trial with carotenoid-rich foods," *Carcinogenesis* 18 (1997): 1847–1850.

Reddy VN, Giblin FJ, Lin L-R, et al., "The effect of aqueous humor ascorbate on ultraviolet-B-induced DNA damage in lens epithelium," *Investigative Ophthalmology and Visual Science* 39 (1998): 344–350.

Robinson K, Arheart K, Refsum H, et al., "Low circulating folate and vitamin B_6 concentrations," *Circulation* 97 (1998): 437–443.

Sarkar A, Basak R, Bishayee A, et al., "B-carotene inhibits rat liver chromosomal aberrations and DNA chain break after a single injection of diethylnitrosamine," *British Journal of Cancer* 76 (1997): 855–861.

Simon JA, Grady D, Snabes MC, et al., "Ascorbic acid supplement use and the prevalence of gallbladder disease," *Journal of Clinical Epidemiology* 51 (1998): 257–265.

Sinatra ST, "Coenzyme Q_{10}: a vitamin therapeutic nutrient for the heart with special application in congestive heart failure," *Connecticut Medicine* 61 (1997): 707–711.

Stephens NG, Parsons A, Schofield PM, et al., "Randomised controlled trial of vitamin E in patients with coronary disease: Cambridge Heart Antioxidant Study (CHAOS), *Lancet* 347 (1996): 781–786.

Thomas MK, Lloyd-Johnes DM, Thadhani RI, et al., "Hypovitaminosis D in medical inpatients," *New England Journal of Medicine* 338 (1998): 777–783.

Suggested Readings and Resources

Below are listed several recommended sources of information on vitamins and your health.

Literature

Balch JF and Blach PA. *Prescription for Nutritional Healing*, second edition. Garden City Park, NY: Avery Publishing Group, 1997.

Challem J and Dolby V. *Homocysteine: The Secret Killer*. New Canaan, CT: Keats, 1997.

Huemer RP and Challem J. *The Natural Health Guide to Beating the Supergerms*. New York: Pocket Books, 1997.

Lieberman S and Bruning N. *The Real Vitamin and Mineral Book*. Garden City Park, NY: Avery Publishing Group, 1997.

Web (Internet) Sites

Medline (for specific medical journal abstracts):
http://www.nlm.nih.gov/databases/ freemedl.
html

The Nutrition Reporter (for summaries of research):
http://www.jackchallem.com

VERIS Research Information Service (for abstracts of antioxidant research):
http://www.veris-online.org

Index